# While I Wait

# My Journey Through Infertility

Anita J. Shaw

Title ID: 7747290
ISBN-13: 978-1979257725

# DEDICATION

I dedicate this book to my girls.

To Abigail, for stretching my faith. You are giving me a new experience of motherhood like I have never known before.

To Darlene Dellinger, for the gift of writing. I still remember the first poem you had published. For your love and for your persistence, thank you.

To my sisters, Sametra, Tameka, and Angel. I love you.  You have made me a protector. I only hope to make you proud and be an example worth following.

# CONTENTS


Dedication iii

Introduction 7

1 The Sound of Babies 10

2 We Changed Our Minds 13

3 Watching the Time Pass By 17

4 My Fertility Process 29

5 Men Struggle Too 42

6 Testing My Marriage 49

7 My Faith 59

8 For This Child, I Prayed 64

9 Dear Family and Friends 72

10 The Promise 80

11 Prayer 86

12   Poem: Passing Season          91

13   Acknowledgements             95

14   Resources                    97

15   Bibliography                 98

16   About the Author             99

# **Introduction**

My battle with infertility is not a story that belongs to me alone, but a parallel of women all over the world. I echo that it is not always easy to start a family. *While I Wait - My Journey Through Infertility* is for every woman that has struggled to conceive and/or give birth. My words are for every woman who searched and researched for answers but ended up with the question why. I have written for the woman who thought they were over the battle, but she miscarried or she gave birth to an angel. This is for the women who blamed herself for not being able to conceive or she was publically shamed for not hitting a "social mile marker."

I have written this for the man who needs to know how to support his woman as she goes through one of the hardest times of her life. These words are for the man who has infertility problems and silently deals with the guilt and shame; he doesn't know what he should do about it. This book is for the woman that hasn't given up hope that one day she could be a mother. To the one who has given up hope, I write to give you back the hope that was slowly stolen from you. As you read, it is alright to release or cry. Give yourself permission to feel. Do me a favor, do not stay in that place. You need to push through and finish. There is hope. I want to show you there is victory in this journey.

I fought the fight of infertility for just shy of five years. Every feeling you have felt, I have probably felt it. It was not always a smooth ride, but I never gave up. Come and share my testimony, my failures, and my victory. You have been waiting on this baby for too long; I want to share some ways that can make the waiting easier. My journey will show you that you are not alone. Often times we can lose ourselves in this process since infertility is a hard obstacle to face. We can forget who we are, what we stand for, and what is important to us. I want to reveal to you that you can still be you until God blesses you with your heart's desires. I want you to find victory, hope, and a path to joy.

Infertility is becoming more and more prevalent in today's society; an unspoken plague that is sweeping through our nation. Most people don't speak about it, and they carry the burden alone. According to CDC in 2017, 12% of women from ages 15-44 have problems conceiving or they have problems carrying a baby to full term (www.cdc.gov/reproductivehealth/index). If you have never experienced infertility, chances are that you are connected to someone that is challenged by it. Allow this book to be a tool for you to assist them along the way. Let's talk about it more. No one should deal with this alone. Once I decided to open my mouth about what my husband and I were dealing with, I found out that I was connected to other people who were having infertility issues as well. The knowledge that I was not alone was a relief. It was helpful knowing that I could share my feelings and medical treatment with people who understood just what I was going through; being able to communicate was a saving grace for me.

# Chapter 1

## *The Sound of Babies*

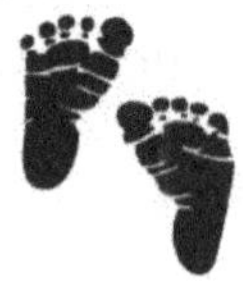

Chime, Chime, Chime.  This is the first sound I hear as I search for my temporary desk in the business office of the hospital. Someone called out of work, and I was their backup. I asked the receptionist where the Medicaid office was located. "Make a right past this office, and it is the second door on the left. Are you filling in for Monica today?" asked the receptionist. Yes, I (Interrupted again by the loud Chime, Chime, Chime - I paused) am. She could tell I was a bit confused about the tune on the intercom, so she said, "Oh that signifies another baby being born in the hospital. I have grown so accustomed to it that I barely hear it now," said the receptionist. I bid her thanks as I walked towards the office.

My stomach was in knots pondering how many babies have been born since I got there; how many were born before I came; and how many more times would I hear that chiming tune for the remainder of the workday. Chime, Chime, Chime. The sound was more pronounced now that I knew what it symbolized. This sound is torture!  While this sound would bring up warm and fuzzy feelings to any other person, the chimes seemed to mock me. It was definitely a distraction during my workday. All I could think about was the difference between the women upstairs and me. Why had God not chosen to bless me with this child yet? What did I do to deserve this? Was I just not ready to have another child? Working back up was usually an easy task, but this time it became rather emotionally taxing.

So it's been just shy of five years since my husband and I embarked on our journey to childbirth. Starting out, we had no idea that it would be a journey. We just thought we could plan to have a baby and it would happen according to plan. According to the birds and bees story that was told by adults, the equation is easy: take a guy and a girl, then zoom boom, and then there is a baby. The formula seemed so simple, foolproof even. Heck, I knew a bunch of people who popped out lots of babies anytime they wanted. Even when they were not trying. Somehow, my bird and bee had a blockage, or dysfunction. We have had difficulty having children and we have been trying everything.

Undetermined Infertility is the diagnosis that sits on the top of my discharge papers at the doctor's office. Infertility, is this a real issue? No one in my family has had trouble having kids. The women in my family could become pregnant if you look at them too long. I did not know anyone with this problem. I didn't even know it was a problem until it was my problem. This journey has been packed with surprises, faith, tears, fears, prayer, trials, but greatest of all persistence.

# CHAPTER 2

## *We Changed our Minds*

Most little girls imagine their dream job, their dream car and house, their dream guy, her dream wedding, and what she would name all of her children. I dreamed it all. I wrote it down. I was committed to the type of future I wanted. I had a plan and expectation. My life started getting off track a bit around my senior year of college.

I got pregnant my senior year in college to a guy I was barely dating. It was one of the scariest and unpredictable times of my life. For a person who prided herself on planning details, I did not see this one coming. No one in my family could believe this was happening to me since I always had myself together and hit all the right marks. Not only was it a shock to the people that knew me, but I disappointed myself by not sticking to my goals I set for myself. I allowed myself to be distracted. While it was difficult, I managed to make it through the school year. I waddled gracefully across the graduation stage six months pregnant. Ironically, I graduated early from college by six months. I grabbed my Bachelor of Science degree just in time! I had a healthy pregnancy and then I gave birth to a handsome, healthy baby boy again without any complications. His name was Amir and he was my little prince. Seeing my son's face gave me a glow inside.

My son's father and I were not in a committed relationship, so I endured the life of a single parent for a while. I did not have much family support locally, so I did the best I could raising this new joy in my life. This is not a sad story though because I made it through that with the grace and mercy of God. Now all the events in my life did not go exactly as planned, but I managed to get my life back on a track I could be proud of.

The culmination of what I wanted in a husband was in a list that I made years ago. Despite my flaws and mistakes, God still blessed me with the man of my dreams. Actually, I received more than I asked for when he arrived. Literally, God exceeded the list I had written out. My husband was over qualified. He not only loved me but he accepted my full package, meaning my son and I. Now I could go back to dreaming…. "White fence, nice house, dream cars, 2.5 kids, and they lived happily ever after."

As a couple, we discussed having more children. We were on the same page with how many children we felt we could handle. When we were engaged, we concluded waiting to have children so that we could spend more time with one another focusing on our relationship. We had to adjust to moving in together and later we wanted to do some traveling. On the night of our wedding, we seemed to change our tune. I don't know if it was the beautiful ceremony, the red rose petals on the Aloft hotel bed, the twinkle in each other's eyes, but something changed our minds that night. As we starred at each other, we joked that it was baby-making time! Somehow, that turned into a real conversation and decision to start making a baby (although not too much talking went on!). It was official; we would start on our wedding night. At this time, I didn't give a thought to what time of the month it was, my cycle, ovulation, or anything else that made scientific sense. I just wanted a baby, and all I knew is that would take us making love that night!

Not for a moment did I believe that it would be a challenge for myself, for my husband, and for my marriage. We figured in a few weeks we would be able to take a test and receive some results. We knew that our family would be expanding soon. On the honeymoon in Playa Del Carmen Mexico, we worked in excess to ensure that whatever babies did not make it on consecration night, made it on this honeymoon trip. We had fun to say the least.

# Chapter 3

## *Watching the time Pass*

We were now in marital bliss, yes newlyweds. We have just experienced one of the most intimate occasions of our lives. We were in love and showing it every chance we got. There was not a care in the world. We knew that we wanted to have a baby. We figured if we just did the "Grown Up" (You know- having sex) it would happen. It was game time. We would go at it every day, sometimes multiple times a day. Our logic was, the more sex we have, the greater our chances would be. Moreover, it was fun, so we did not mind. Now at this time, we did not know anything about optimizing our chances by following my ovulation cycle. What we did believe was that lots of sex would lead us having some signs and symptoms of our new arrival soon.

A month passed, my cycle came on. No big deal. There is always next month. I am sure it takes other people a month or two to have a baby. I can wait another month no problem. Month two then three passed by. There was still no reason to be alarmed, but the anxiety started to build up. It was very early in the game. Everyone around us was excited about our new marriage and excited that we wanted to have a baby soon. They expected results just as we did. Every month friends and family members would do a visual examination of my figure to make sure I did not have "The Glow" or "A Baby Bump." The spectating of the crowd surrounding our life was a reminder to me almost daily there was a desire of mine that had not yet arrived.

We have to be careful when we have goals and dreams that other people's expectations don't become a barrier. Other people's expectations can mirror an alternate reality in a way. Be careful not to be driven by other people's desires and plans more than your own. Your vision can be endangered due to the feelings of others. Other people's expectations can cause you added pressure on top of your anxiety in any given situation. Other's expectation can direct more attention to you. For example, if my neighbor expects me to be pregnant by month three and she makes it known every time she sees me. She may also bring my lack of conceptions to other people's attention with her constant visual and vocal expression of her expectations. This causes more pressure. All eyes are on me to produce something that I obviously have no control over.

## Months 6-12 of Waiting

Now we are getting a little antsy. Where is this bundle of Joy? This should have happened by now. I went to my primary care doctor for a regular checkup, and while I was there, I shared my concerns. We have been trying for six months now and nothing, no baby. I asked the doctor, at what point should I become concerned and ready to take other action? The doctor assured me that the worry mark should be at year number one. Most couples conceive within one year if there are no issues. She let me know that it was still early and that I should just keep trying. She let me know that since we were both young and my first pregnancy was without complication that we should not have an issue. This news was very reassuring. It is still early, nothing is wrong. We just needed to keep trying. She also offered the advice to keep up with my ovulation and make sure that we are having sex on those days. Trying is fun! No problem, we can do that.

So we brought some ovulation kits at the drug store and kept trying. No major pressure. Just more aware of what we were trying to accomplish when we would have sex. I started keeping charts in my calendar book of my menstrual cycle starting at month seven. I also started to do some research on what to do in order to conceive faster. We researched which positions were more effective for childbirth; In hindsight, I don't know that any of the positions were helpful. We tried changing our diet: we added more greens, more water, pomegranate juice, berries, fish, etc. I tried elevating my knees to my chest after we had sex to help the sperm travel to where they needed to be. All the while, those family, friends, co-workers, and church family did not cease in reminding me that they expected a baby soon. At times, it almost felt as if I had an obligation to them to produce. The word Produce, so industrial. A word that simulates one putting in work. This is what the stress of trying to make a baby started to become- Production.

In some industries, there are manufacturing assembling lines. On occasion, I felt like my uterus was on that assembly line and was up for evaluation; ultimately falling below company standards because there was no product at the end. My husband and I were working on it, but there was nothing to show for the hard work as of yet. This was no fun. Now I notice everyone else was popping babies off the assembly lines as if they worked at the Ford Company, except the product was wrapped in blue or pink. Some of these people did not want a baby, did not plan for a baby, or frankly were not fit to care for any children (DSS exist for a reason, some people fit in this category). Meanwhile, I craved a baby.

We have been waiting. We have exhausted our efforts and knowledge trying. One emotion after another. One disappointment after another. Everything in me could not stop wanting, so that meant I could not stop waiting until I saw what I was expecting. I knew that God's word never fails and I knew he would not leave nor forsake me. In the spiritual realm, we began to praise God in advance for our blessing. I praised God for what I did not have because I knew that it was on its way. I did not know when, but I praised and thanked him for this baby anyway. Not only did I take this disposition but my family took it on as well. I began to thank him morning, noon, and night for what was coming. I began to pray even harder.

## Year 2

By this point, I thought something might be wrong with me. Was there something wrong with my husband? According to the doctors, after one year we should be concerned. We were now in year two and we did not have the results of conceiving a baby. After year one of trying to conceive, you are classified as having infertility issues. It was at this point that I began feeling like seeking out a specialist would be in our best interest.

## My Faith Walk

While all of the life was going on, I still believed that God would make a way out of no way. While medical alternatives were being considered, I also considered what I needed to do with my faith walk with God. I began to spend even more time with God while I was going through this journey. I prayed more. I prayed more not only because I needed God to bless me with this baby, but also because I needed God to help me maintain. Meaning, I still was a mother, a wife, I still had a job to go to, I was still a sister, I was still a friend, and I was in school obtaining my master's degree at the time. I had obligations. Part of my prayer to God would just ask him to help keep and guide me. I needed to perform in every area of my life with the same level of excellence that I did before I knew I wanted a baby. This desire that I had could not stop me from living my life. We prayed. Our prayers became more and more desperate towards God as time passed by. I was begging the Lord to bless us. I prayed more now more than ever, I needed to know God more. Spending time with God in prayer and spending time in the word of God is the only way to know him better.

In the spiritual realm, we also began to sow seeds of Faith. The bible speaks of sowing and reaping. I truly believe that if I give/pour into good ground, I shall reap a harvest so great that I will not have room enough to receive. Throughout my time of waiting on my baby to manifest naturally, my husband and I would sow seeds. For those that may not be familiar with this concept, there were times my husband and I would give a specific amount of money and sow it (in other words give it) to our ministry, our leader, or often times even to a stranger in need. We learned that we must always have a destination in mind when sowing, so our hearts and minds would be on what we needed from God when we were giving. This seeding is not to be confused with tithing or offering, but it was an extra offering to God. We called our seed by name every time we gave, hoping that what we gave was acceptable, and that it ultimately would gain God's attention. We sowed a few times over the course of the years, and we believed that he would answer our prayers.

Praising was another part of our waiting process. We gave God an advance praise. What is that? We praised him as if we already had our gift. I can give you an example of what it might look like so you can have a visual. If someone came up to me and said here is 5 million dollars, the way I would start running and shouting across the room. The way I would probably cry and fall to my knees in gratitude, this is the type of praise that we would offer up to God. We just needed God to know that we believed in his promise to us and that we knew he would bless us when the time was right. As much as this advanced praise was a blessing for him, it was a release for my husband and I. At times, praising God with everything you have lifts a burden off you. It frees you from thinking about what you don't have and it allows you to focus on how amazing God truly is.

## Feelings of Rejection

There are so many emotions that you go through when waiting a long time on whatever God has for you. Especially when it comes to having children. Procreation is what humans were designed to do from the beginning. As a woman, once you have started puberty, you have a monthly reminder of what your body is created to do. Your body starts preparing for childbirth way before a woman decides to have children. Therefore, as I go from month to month waiting on the interruption of this cycle indicating life, I wait. It gives a new meaning to the term cycle. I literally figure out new ways to conceive,  and I to go through the emotional rollercoaster repeatedly.

I went from being excited to have a child and eager to start, to anxiously waiting. There were times when I worried that something was wrong. There were times I wanted to place blame on someone or something. Is it me? Is it my husband? What did I do wrong? Was this is payback for me having a child out of wedlock (in other words having sex and conceiving a baby before I got married). I searched for any reason in my mind to make this make sense. I am a very logical reasoning type of person, and I needed this to make sense. This is the thing, how God chooses to organizes my life does not conceptually need to make sense to me. It is not supposed to. I believe and trust that he knows best.

This did not stop me from being a little resentful and angry with others who did not want any children at all but still managed to conceive. It did not stop me from being in awe of the people who were not expecting children and did not have any plans to expand their family, but ended up with children anyway. I was most disheartened with those parents who chose not to be parents by means of abortion or choosing to give their children up for adoption. I mean no disrespect to anyone who made this decision, but my desperation made me long for what I could not have in ways I could not imagine.

These strong emotions come from the fact that I lay begging God daily for a child. I was not one of those people who hated everyone that conceived because I was not pregnant yet (despite what some may have thought about me). There were people I was rooting for to get pregnant. Then I went back to thoughts of rationalizing. I would say that maybe it is not my time and God knows best. Although it sounds like a cliché, I really knew that these things were the truth. Knowing that if I wait on the Lord and renew my strength, that he would mount me up. Victory is on the way. So while I wait, I will serve him.

I know that God loves me. He has blessed me before, even when I did not deserve it. I know that his word is true and he cannot lie, but waiting is often what we hate doing. I know that God can and most importantly, I know that he will give me this baby. While you wait on what he has for you, the enemy will try to make you doubt. The enemy will try to steal your joy. Seems like I was invited to more baby showers during this period of my life than I have ever before, which is a hard event to attend given my circumstances. Why is this surrounding me? Because this is what I am waiting on. People come to me almost daily to ask me about having a baby as if I could literally choose the day I conceive. On occasion, the same person multiple times in a week. If they only knew the sword that it shoved into my heart with each question. Or how every now and then I faught back the tears with a smile. If they only knew, I went to bed thinking about conceiving and woke up with it on my mind. If they knew that intimacy with my husband was full of pressure and stress because of my thoughts of possible disappoint from not having a baby.

There were so many nights I prayed and cried. Most times, I believed I was strong enough to handle it, other times I had to look into my husband's eyes and think about not being able to give him what he desired most. I felt like I let him down. Seeing my husband pray over my stomach, even when he thought I wasn't aware. The look of disappointment when he sees a monthly Kotex wrapper in the trash. The void I feel as a woman not being able to do what I was designed to do is a hard feeling to bare.

I just want you to know that if infertility is what you're struggling with, I have probably felt every raw emotion that you have felt. There is no sugar coating, these feelings are real and some days were a battle. If you are a believer, you are not exempt from feeling. Misfortune and trial may hit you in life, and you will feel it. The key is not to allow your feelings to run your life. Pick yourself up and find a way to refocus, and move forward one day at a time. We will explore some step to help you get through as we navigate through the chapters. While this process was not always easy, everyday was not a battle for me.

# Chapter 4

# My Fertility Process

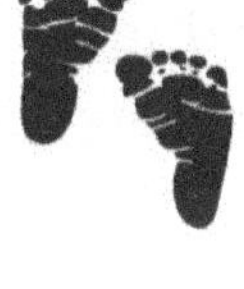

I concluded that I needed to attempt another avenue since I tried everything that I possibly could. I have waited, prayed, and praised. I went to my primary care physician. I tried multiple sexual positions and increased the quantity of times we would have sex. I charted my menstrual cycle. I cried and prayed some more. I seeded. I changed my diet. Everything that I could do, I was doing it, and it was not enough, I needed assistance.

There had to be someone who specialized in this. I did not know anyone I could gather advice from, so I did some research and found the best fertility specialist in the south. She just happened to be local to my area. Finding a doctor was easy; thinking about bringing this idea up to my husband was another. I just imagined him saying let's wait it out, that's too expensive, or just no; but he didn't. I believe that this whole experience had him just as beat too. Choosing to go to a fertility doctor just gave us a second wind. We figured we would go to a consultation and see what our options were and most importantly, what it would cost. If we liked what we heard and if it did not cost us a kidney, we would do it. If we did not like it or it was out of our price range, then at least, we can say we tried. During this entire process, we have been giving our best shot.

We set up our consult and immediately fell in love with our doctor. She was empathetic to our situation, knowledgeable, nice, she gave us hope, she was realistic, and she let us know what our process would be. She was warm and she understood how fragile the situation was for us. Next, we had a meeting with the financial counselor who explained to us how much the process would cost. She also went over the different options we had to pay for it and how to maximize our Blue Cross and Blue Shield insurance plans throughout the process. When we left, we left satisfied with the consult.

Let me share three main takeaway points from our consult. The first is that it is ok to go to a doctor/ specialist for help. Too often we know we need help and we just sit there and take it. In life when we see that our circumstances in life are not getting better, don't accept that. You can not stay in that rut; there are too many resources available for you to be in the position you are in, suffering. No matter what rut you are in, in any area of your life, don't settle. No matter what you think of my tactics to get pregnant up until this point, what you cannot say is that I did not try. Secondly, consulting with a specialist/doctor is just that, a consult; it does not commit you to anything. Consults give you information so that you can make an informed decision concerning your specific situation. Acquire the information. In our despair, we make all the hypothetical situations in the world. We assume how things will go, assume what it will cost, but we don't actually go through with any of the steps. GO FIND OUT! Finding out is the cheapest part of the process, I promise.

Lastly, I want you to know that the fertility process is not a cookie cutter process, so the prices vary, and the process varies for every couple. The procedures or lack thereof may vary from couple to couple. Do not let finances be the reason that you do not check out your options, there are all types of financing options and payment plans that you can check out. When you go to the fertility doctor or your primary care physician, remember that there is no magic bullet. Finding a solution for you may be a medical process of elimination to solve your problem.

The reason prices for the fertility process vary is because it depends on which doctor you see, the insurance you have or lack thereof, the test you need, the procedures you need or lack thereof, the amount of time it takes you to get pregnant, the options available for your particular situation, and so on. So many variables are involved that make your situation unique, it would be difficult to give you a price on how much it would cost to solve your infertility issues. I am unsure about the amount we truly paid from start to finish because we paid it as we went along and as situations came up.

Tyrone and I were reasonable about what we could afford and when it was feasible to do so. Nevertheless, it was affordable and we did not finance it. We figured it out along the way because we wanted it. Occasionally that meant putting off a test or procedure until the following month, but we got it all done. It was not nearly as expensive as I had imagined. You will never know what your process will be like and what your price will be like if you don't try. We buy $20k cars, $200k houses, pay God knows what on college tuition (some of those refund checks don't even go toward education - to tell the truth), and hundreds or thousands on vacations. Surely having a baby is worth it. I am not telling you to live beyond your means here or to go broke reproducing; I am saying if you have been having trouble conceiving for some time or your health is working against you, just find out if this is a viable option for you. Be open to working it out.

My consult went well. My husband and I were not previously financially prepared to take this on, so we had to be smart about how we approached this. We got a plan together and started our process. I can remember the first time we entered the room for an ultrasound. I left with such hope. I saw my healthy follicles. More than the average woman. My plentiful eggs had a great shape and size. My Uterus was a great shape and size, and it was in a great position. Thank God! Some great news, some hope. Healthy potential babies are just laying around waiting for something to "pop off." Although the ultrasound was just the beginning, it gave me more confidence than I've had in a while. God will find a way to give you a little boost in the mist of what you are going through. I needed that boost, my husband needed that boost, and more importantly, our marriage needed that news.

Over the course of 2 years, I saw the fertility specialist. It does not have to take this long for everyone; again, every situation is unique. I took some breaks in between for my body, mind, and finances. During these two years, I gave many blood samples. Sometimes my poor little veins would just give out; I imagine they were tired too. The specialist used blood to check what is going on in your body good or bad, monitor my hormone levels, checked for pregnancy, and I am sure they checked and monitored a host other bodily functions.

At first, it seemed like they could not pinpoint any real problem. Since my egg count was high and something was off in my blood work, it was a possibility that I might have PCOS. PCOS stands for Polycystic Ovary Syndrome. This is a problem in which a woman's hormones are out of balance. It can cause problems with your periods and make it difficult to get pregnant. I did not really meet the entire criteria for it, but it could explain why I had so many eggs. Well at this point, coming up with a problem to solve is better than the unknown. So I began to take Metformin on a regular basis and changed my diet and exercise habits dramatically. This meant that everyone in my family had changes in their diets also.

I took a hysterosalpingogram test in which they looked at my fallopian tubes and uterus. This test found a potential problem, but lead to another test. I then took a saline sonohysterogram. This showed an endometrial polyp inside of my uterus. While this polyp was not harmful to me, it would not be a suitable environment for a baby to grow in and it had to go. This discovery lead to surgery, a polypectomy. Essentially this was the scrapping of my uterus. Even though I found a problem that I could fix, at that time it was not great news. I began to think of all the times I thought I was pregnant, but then it turned out to be nothing. Well, in fact, it might have been something; maybe the polyp just snuffed it out before we had a chance to really know. That made me feel awful. Although I had no way of knowing I had polyps in my uterus, I felt guilty for not knowing. Moreover, what If I have this surgery and it still does not solve our problem. Some people take surgeries lightly, but every time you go under anesthesia with sharp instruments, it is a huge risk. You are totally dependent on someone dilly dabbing around with sharp objects while you are heavily medicated and unconscious. Scary. Oh well, I had to do what I had to do. At the end of the day, I would do everything in my power to give this baby the best shot. I decided to have the surgery. My husband was by my side the whole way. The doctor that performed my surgery said I would not feel much of anything afterwards, and I could go back to work, but I had loads pressure in my stomach for about a week. I was still able to function, but it was just uncomfortable. I took one day off from work to rest. I preached a sermon three days later and pressed my way through the discomfort. I still went to work and went on through all the other daily activities.

There could be no baby making talk after the surgery due to my healing period. I needed a break anyway. I took a few more months from the specialist just to get my head back in the game. During this resting period, I still took my medication, vitamins, did my PCOS eating, etc. I still had my body prepared for a little one just in case. I still believed that God would keep his promise to me.

Finally, I went back to the fertility doctor. All test were complete and now it was time for a plan of attack. We decided to proceed with an IUI. This is intrauterine insemination where a doctor inserts the sperm directly into the uterus. This helps the sperms not have to travel so far, biologically they already know where to go; this process just helps them not to detour. Since I had numerous healthy eggs and my spouse had many healthy sperm, we did not need a donor.

For this procedure, we had to prepare the best egg for the best sperm. This entire process was very time sensitive. After carefully tracking my cycle the last few month, my doctor handed me a calendar and it appeared my cycle had a booked schedule. On certain days of my cycle, I had to take medication. On other days, I had to take medication and inject Gonal in my stomach with a needle. The medication would sometimes burn going in during the injections. Not sure if it was my hormones, the medication, or this process in general, but I was more fatigued during this process. After ten days, I would come back in for labs and for monitoring. Then on the right day, I had the IUI. Tyrone gave his fresh sperm sample and they were cleaned and ready to work.

What did the procedure feel like? The best way to describe it is like a pap smear with the exception that you would wait awkwardly afterwards with your legs elevated. You get undressed from bottoms down, get up on the table and place your feet in stirrups, and the doctor sticks a catheter into your vagina to insert the washed sperm from your partner. Tyrone was by my side throughout the process. The whole thing took a few minutes.  Afterwards, I had to lay with my feet elevated for about 10-15 minutes.

I took the remaining of the day to rest, I did not want those babies mixing up too much. We had to wait about two weeks before we knew if the procedure worked. This was the longest two weeks ever, we were so anxious. At some point, I received a call to let me know the result of the IUI. The day we have been anticipating, but the news was not what we were waiting on. After all this time and effort, it failed. I was not pregnant. What a blow! This should have been the fairytale ending, but it was just another chapter in my testimony.

How do I bounce back from this? How will my husband take the news? What do I do next? Before I could figure any of that out, the first thing I did was cry. I asked God what I was supposed to do. I was distraught after all my body has gone through I could not believe we failed. That is what it felt like, failure. For a few days, maybe even weeks after, I was a zombie. I just went through the motions, but I was numb. I have never knowingly lost a child, but I imagine it was a similar feeling at this stage (this is the only way I can describe it).

During that period of waiting for my results, I just knew I was pregnant. All the ingredients were there. When I got the news that there was no baby, I felt like I lost my baby. I mean no disrespect to any woman who has ever had a miscarriage and I do not make light of it. The difference in my loss is that it happened early in the process, which correlates to age-old question of when does life begin. Depending on how you answer that question, would be the difference in your level of empathy for this early loss of life. Mentally and emotionally to me, there was no difference. I felt like I lost a baby. I grieved.

People around me had no idea of the battle I faced from day to day, but during this period surely they noticed my grief. It showed. I don't apologize for it. It did not stop me from performing any of my day-to-day tasks, but I grieved, I did not stay in this place. I understood that I needed to press forward.

I could not keep going this way emotionally. I am the product of a failed suicide attempt as a teenager, so I don't take acute depression lightly even if this was situational. Not long after receiving the results, my husband and I spoke with our Pastor about our failed procedure and the process we went through. He gave us some encouragement. He did not sugar coat our pain, but he also knew our level of faith in God and did not let our faith off the hook. He commanded the faith we had inside of us to stand up and to stand firm. He encouraged us to keep pressing, as he knew and believed with us that this was not the end of our story. He prayed with us. I will not tell you that my countenance instantly changed because it did not. I knew that everything he said was true cause I knew what God's word said. I knew that he promised me this baby. My Pastor was praying with us. I knew that I had back up in the spirit. I knew that he would keep praying until the promise manifested.

I knew that he would keep encouraging me. If you do not have that person in your life for this process, put that on your to do list. Make that your next step in this process. You need people who are going to keep you lifted and encouraged. Remember I told you that I went through days when I was numb and just coasting through each day; those prayers are what kept me. Those prayers kept me from crashing into another car due to my mind being elsewhere, kept me working when I felt like I just wanted to be buried under the covers, it kept me involved with my son although I wish I did not feel like being anybody's anything. Those prayers moved me right past that stage until I could turn the page on those feelings.

After some time, my husband and I decided to try again. We saved up and tried it again. We prayed up and tried again. Were we insane? Maybe a little. What made us try again? The simple answer is Faith. I know it did not work the first time, but there was a chance it could work again. My bible commands us to multiply, and I saw the miracles of a woman in the bible who had trouble conceiving and conceived such as Hannah and Sarah. I know that God wants me to prosper in all things as long as I prosper in him. I know how faithful I have been to God and in ministry. I know that God promised me this child. I know that there is no biological reason that the doctors have seen that would keep me from conceiving at this point. I cannot stop desiring to conceive a child, I TRIED. Again, there was a drive inside of me that would not allow me to stop trying to conceive. I could not be afraid to trust God. If you are a believer, believe. You must believe when it is easy and believe when it is tough.

We did our second IUI July 27, 2015. Same rigorous, tight scheduled process. We decided to go in with just as much Faith as we did the first go around. It was not easy, we had to repeat all the steps. We had to save up some money to pay for the procedure, I had do all the medication treatment according to the schedule, I had to endure injections, Tyrone gave another sperm sample, and we did the insemination procedure when the time was right. When the IUI process was over, we had the awkward wait for result again. Then, we received the call. There was a baby this time; it worked.

# Chapter 5

# Men Struggle Too

We cannot assume that a couple struggling with conception automatically means that it must be the woman's fault. Men struggle with infertility issues also. Some male fertility issues are equally as serious as female issues and may result in them not being able to produce children just like women. A host of the issues can be resolved with some treatment. In order to resolve the issues, there must be an acknowledgement that there is an issue and then seek out some medical treatment. There are four main causes of infertility in males: a pituitary disorder, a gonad disorder, or unknown cause which are where 40-50% of the problems stem from (www.Americanpregnancy.org/infertility/male-infertility). The unknown is the greatest disturbance for obvious reasons; there is no known problem to fix. The point is men struggle with producing too.

My husband Tyrone had his own issues with infertility. Like me, he was excited to begin the baby-making mission. He had no idea what we were in for. Just like a great deal of couples we just thought when we decided to have kids, it would happen. Once we reached a certain point in trying to conceive, he started to think our inability to conceive was his fault. His rationale was that because I had already conceived a child without complication that he must be the cause. As a wife, I tried to assure him that we needed to find out for sure what the cause was and that we should not jump to any conclusions. I always tried to be supportive of him throughout this process by letting him know no matter what the issues are; we would work through them together. Besides he was young, he did not smoke or drink; he was healthy, he worked out regularly, and his diet was good. There was a great chance that his sperm was in tip-top shape.

The same way he expressed his excitement about having kids with me often, he expressed his concerns with me when it started taking longer than expected. He did not mind telling me about all his aspirations when the baby was born. He shared his hopes that he would have a baby girl who would melt his heart as well as his pockets. He already had a picturesque future imagined before the baby was even formed. He also told me about times when he was worried. He was burdened by the possibility that he would be the hold up of our blessing. He never let his concern show too much. He would somehow look like he believed it would happen. He did not let it slow him down in his daily life.

Every healthy change I made to give us better chances at conceiving, he was happy to make the change as well. He tried the dieting, exercising more, taking multivitamins daily, and every other wildly idea I could come up with. He also gave up coffee, caffeine drinks, and hot baths, which are all bad for sperm health. Prior to knowing we would be attending the fertility specialist, I suggested he take a natural herb called Maca Root. This was supposed to boost his sperm count. He was on board for the super sperm idea. We did some research, and soon he was popping those pills like candy. He took the pills for a few weeks, and no baby came. Physically we noticed the change in the volume of his sperm, but we don't really know what the quality of the sperm was because we didn't know any better at this point. We had no idea if taking Maca Root hurt us or helped us, but it did not get us the results we wanted. One of the first steps in the male fertility process if checking the sperm. In order to do this, you give a sample for semen analysis. When we went to the fertility doctor, we had to give them a couple of babies in a cup so they could check them out. I say we, but really, I had nothing to do with this process. It was all on him to get those babies in that cup. Since this was not really his thing, this part of the process was uncomfortable for him in that little room.

When he had his first semen analysis at the fertility clinic, the numbers were decent but not impressive, but the number is not the only variable that matters. They also look at shape (morphology) and mobility. His test showed that he was below average in mobility and morphology. All of these factors determine how much sperm is in the race and how many are able to go the distance. This was a low blow for Tyrone. These results confirmed everything that he was already feeling about it being his fault that we have not gotten pregnant yet. He immediately blocked out any chance that the issues could be with the both of us and started blaming himself even more. He shared his disappointments with me freely. It was emasculating news. Seeing his face while he talked about the results made me feel helpless. I did not know what caused this problem or why this was happening, but to see him in this place emotionally was challenging.

If you know my husband Tyrone, you know that he lights up any room that he walks into. He is always upbeat, loves to make jokes, always smiling, and just an all-around easygoing guy. This infertility issue was standing in the way of him having what his heart longs for, a baby. Not only that, he blames my heartache of wanting a child on himself. He had his family, our future, and his manhood all stacked on his shoulders. No matter what I said to him, it was never enough to convince him that it was not his fault.

As devastating this news was, he still held a standard in his duties as a father, a husband, at work, at church, and in the community. He continued to be an amazing father to our son Amir. He still made sure that he not only provided for our son, but that he still made time for quality time together doing what interest Amir like going to the indoor jump place, going to the movies, or just playing games. He still helped Amir with homework and attended functions at school. He still preached at church and upheld his duties as a minister and Elder. He still worked hard at his job and maintained a level of integrity and leadership that he brags on often.

An astounding segment of Tyrone's life that I have witnessed was seeing him give himself to children that needed him. Children in our neighborhood and the community know him by name. They all come up to him while he is working in the garage or while he is in the yard just to talk. Occasionally they came to him because they needed a part fixed on their bikes; other times parents called him on the phone because their children needed some guidance from a father figure. He remained a mentor to many children at a time when he had trouble producing a biological child of his own. He did not let that stop him from pouring into the lives of others. Seeing Tyrone give his heart to others and seeing him power through adversity, made me proud as a wife.

After the less than desirable sperm analysis results, the doctor insisted that Tyrone stop the Maca Root all together and she prescribed a medication called Clomid. Clomid is supposed to improve his sperm count and help to balance out any hormone imbalances. The problem that Tyrone faced sounds bad, but it is not the end of the world. He took the prescribed medication consistently and as directed. Over the course of two years, Tyrone had to have about ten semen specimens taken for analysis. His number, mobility, and morphology improved with the use of Clomid. One of his results was so high he was walking around as if he had super powers. This definitely improved his confidence and gave him a new outlook on our problem. We began to see our infertility as something to conquer one rung at a time instead of a massive ladder of disappointment. Throughout out the remainder of the fertility process, he just had to show up, give sperm when needed, and support me.

# Chapter 6

# Testing My Marriage

When you fall in love, that is the easy part. It's all fun and roses. I was literally guided by those butterflies in my stomach when I met my husband. I was moved by just seeing him. This made getting to know him sweatless. Something happens after the butterflies, it's called Life. Now that does not mean that the fun and roses goes away, but sometimes you must put in work to make roses and fun. The problems I faced with infertility had a significant effect on my marriage over time.

At first, it was just fun to imagine the thought of having a baby together. Who would the baby look like? Who would the baby act like? We would imagine the outfits we could dress him or her in. We wondered whose toes the baby would have. Besides the hypothetical scenarios, it was fun trying to make the baby at first. We were young, and a chance to be intimate often was a high. After about a year and a half, something was different and the high faded. It has nothing to do with attraction or performance, but the pressure of this baby. Intimacy became an effort. We realized that we had to try and try hard. If you think that just means more sex, well you would be half right. Between the regimented sex, the restrictions that changed our lifestyles, the doctors' visits, the medication, the medication side effects, the charting, the diet changes, work, family life, church, and all the other entities that surrounded us at times; making a baby became a full time job. It was no fun. Don't get me wrong, I love my husband, and I know that he loves me; but that pressure coming from all directions makes it hard to be free. Because there is an ovulation window, you must make sure you have sex on certain days. With our crazy work schedules, that was not always convenient, nor was it sexy.

Besides our work schedule, we added other variables to our marriage to make it stressful like googling. At times, just knowing more adds stress and that's where Google comes into play. When we first noticed that this baby was taking a long time, we started by just googling tips on what could help us conceive. This changed our dieting and exercise habits at first. Next, we found out that Tyrone should not drink his morning coffees due to it causing low sperm count. We also both cut back on sugars and sodas, we added a weekly serving of pomegranate juice, we added prenatal vitamins, we added more green leafy foods, we added more proteins, and we added more berries. We also increased water intake dramatically. Not too bad right? We should have been doing these things anyway. No big deal.

The next level was the charting. Charting is keeping track of your fertility cycle. This can be done with pen and paper or it can be done electronically; they have free apps that you can download on your phone to make it easier. To start, when you document when your cycle starts and when it stops, and track when you are ovulating. You also need track each time you have sex, track your cervical position, track your basal temperature each morning, and tracking your cervical fluid (other charting methods may have you track some additional items as well). This may not seem like a task, but I did this on and off for the better part of three years. Three years is what makes it feel like a task. While this particular task was not one we shared together, it still added to stress in my marriage. It became a part of a list of items that I had to endure that my spouse did not, and it caused a bit resentment. When you add a chart to anything fun, it takes the fun out of it.

Charting lets you know exactly when you should have sex to maximize your chances at conception. There is a small window in the month when a woman is most fertile, and you must have sex during this window come rain, sleet, or snow. Pressure!!! This means, you having sex when you are in the mood and when you are not in the mood. Not that I did not enjoy it, but after a time it was no longer for enjoyment. We had a job to do, procreate. We would often joke to each other that we would use each other like a piece of meat! Well, that was true often, but we were both content with that. Sometimes that meant those long sexy sessions with all the bells and whistles were reduced down to a quickie so that we can be sure to make this window.

Let me give you a scenario of what this means for us. For example, if Tuesday is our highest chance to conceive that month we must make sure we have sex that day. Well, if Tyrone is on night shift the night before, that means he wouldn't get off from work and get home until about 5:45 to 6:00 am. I get up at 5: 45 am to get our son ready for school. I start getting myself ready for work at about 6:30. Our son leaves the house to get on the bus at 6:30 am, and I need to make sure that he leaves on time. Between 7:00 and 7:10, I need to be out of the house. My husband has usually put his gear away, showered, and is in bed by 6:40 am after working a 13-hour shift. I work for 8 hours and drive in 30 minutes of traffic to meet him with our son since he has to be off to work again. There is about a 15-20 min window in this day for us to possibly meet this window. Not every day was this hectic, but it was a normal part of our week when we had to work and Amir had school.

Going to the doctors also caused pressure. Our primary care physicians just could not figure out why two young, healthy individuals could not conceive. It was even stranger that I had given birth prior without complications to a healthy baby. Going to the fertility specialist turned out to be the best decision we ever made for our family, but it did not always feel that way. The frequency of the appointments, the money we were not prepared to spend, the test, the medication, the constant blood drawing, and the hormones. Just the totality of it all created more stress to our growing desire to conceive. Money and Medication can add pressure to any situation by itself.

Family, friends, and peers did not make it any better for our situation. Just another brick on the heavy load. The insensitive questions and statements that are spoken in light are sometimes hurtful. After a long day of dieting restrictions, charting, yucky gummy prenatal vitamins, doctor visits where I have been poked and prodded; it just not tolerable. I could say the words people say do not matter, but the fact is it does. And when a couple is fighting for a child, it adds fuel to the fire causing additional stress.

Up until this point, I talked about how hard it was. It was only hard at times. I can't give you a percent of the time due to it varying over the years. What I will say is that the good days outweighed the bad days. I will say that having a husband that was also my friend, my prayer partner, and my support made going through this easier. We made each other laugh even when we wanted to cry. We told infertility jokes to each other that would be in poor taste to repeat, but it got us through a tough day. We prayed together. We text each other scriptures throughout the week for encouraged. We still went on dates and found chances to remember why we got married in the first place. We did every step of this process together. If I had to make a diet change, he made one too. If he had to drink more water, I did too. He went to as many doctor visits with me as he could. And of most value, we talked. Proper communication was key in getting through this period.

Talking to each other can often get lost in all the noise of life. There were a lot of moving pieces in our lives at this point, but we talked. We talked about what we wanted, we made a plan, we had steps to get to our goal, and we executed the plan. We talked about our goals, we talked about our bodies, our health, our faith, our failures, he discussed his feelings of failures as a man, and I discussed my feelings of failure as a woman, we talk about what everyone else said about us, we talked about each doctor visit, and we talked about where we stood with each other throughout this process. We did not always communicate perfectly. Maybe this has happened to you before, but occasionally when I speak, he listens but hears something very different from what actually came out of my mouth. This goes both ways. This causes lots of confusion at times, but we found a way to work through that too.

This process is so delicate; you have to talk it through. Every day brings a new challenge, and you need to be in communication to see how you can overcome the challenge.

We knew that the desire that we had was at the forefront of our lives, but it did not consume us. There were other responsibilities in life we needed to tend to. We also knew that what we were already blessed with in life was enough to be grateful for. My husband and I reminded each other about what God has already blessed us with. Every now and then, we would go overboard on loving each other just because it released some of the stress from the situation. He would give me gifts just because, leave me notes in my car that said I love you, or just overwhelm me with extra affection. I likewise would drop off his favorite snack at work unexpectedly, leave a note of love in his sock drawer, or whisper sweet nothings in his ear to leave him thinking about just me. We could not afford to let this process draw a wedge in our marriage, so we made sure we did extra things to show our love to one another to prevent that from happening.

You may say, well my situation is different; there is no way to get through this. You may think that there is no solution for your problem. I would argue that you are not the only one with that unique situation. Someone somewhere has that same issue with infertility that you are having; and with those same variables, they found a way to work it out. You can too. From time to time, we can't think of the answers to our problems on our own, but maybe we know someone that could help us figure it out. My Pastor always tells us that if you don't have what you need or don't understand something, tap into someone else that has what you need. Use your resources. Think of the best movie you have ever seen. Do you have it in mind? That movie took a whole team of people to bring it to fruition. No one person on the team does it all, but there is a whole lot of creative minds tapping into each other to cultivate each other's creativity to form the brilliant production you love. That movie is a classic to you now. Well if you begin to tap into some people and information, a shift can cultivate and change your situation. Every solution to your particular issue may not be ideal, but it may be necessary for your end goal.

Everything we did to our bodies and with our time was for the end goal, a baby. It did not always feel good, taste good, or look good; but it all worked out for our good. Even when I did not understand why I went through what I went through, I knew that it was not for naught. I knew there was purpose. I wanted to give up plenty of days, but my faith would not let me. I knew as long as we kept God first, talked openly with each other, and kept supporting one another we could and would conquer anything.

# Chapter 7

# My Faith

My faith in God is all that I have to stand on. It is all that I know, and it is my foundation. Faith carries me from day to day. I know that God is able to do whatever I need done no matter how big or small. In this situation, I did not have a choice but to wait until the baby came. What I did while I waited was up to me. I knew that God was watching me while I waited to see how I would act. I recognized there were people depending on me to keep it together.

No matter what you are going through, God expects a certain level of kingdom decorum from us. Kingdom decorum is keeping behavior in good taste and propriety according to the word of God. I needed to act as if I believed that this would happen. I also knew that other people in my life were watching me to see how I will act during this difficult time. Whether I realized it or not, someone was always watching me. I did not wallow in a pity party or drown myself in tears daily. I will never stop believing in God, nor would I stop serving him no matter the circumstances. I will not stop caring for my children or my spouse because life has gotten hard. God has been so incredible to me that if he decided to never do another thing, he has already done more than enough for me in my life. He has blessed me beyond measure.

Not for one day did I stay in bed all day due to my circumstances not being favorable. Not one day did I stay home from the job God blessed me with because I was upset. The inability to conceive a baby did not keep me from going to church or from serving God. This situation did not keep me from thanking God daily, praising him, or worshiping him. God inhabits the praise of his people; he deserves it no matter what situation is happening in your life. God's kingdom, God's purpose for my life, and my salvation is more important than any of my desires. Is wanting a baby a valid desire? Yes, it is. I also realized the entire time that God understood just how bad I wanted a baby. He knew that I would not give up. He knew what I was willing to endure to obtain the promise. It was hard. Can you believe him even when it is hard to do so?

Does this mean that I never cried or had a day where I was down? No, I had those days, but I did not stay in that place. I do not allow my circumstances or what people say to keep me in that place. I am blessed and I live a blessed life. I know that I live in the abundance of God right now. I am favor and I shall have everything that my father promised me. I will not tell you that you will get every desire of your heart because some things were not meant for us to have even though we desire them. You ought to trust that God knows best about what you need and when you need it. Do you trust him?

Think about the hardest situation that you have ever experienced in your life and then think about how you escaped it. You realize that it was only God that helped you out of the situation. The baby that I asked him for is a small request compared to that. What you are asking him for may seem like its big to you, but it's easy for God. He is able to do exceedingly and abundantly above all I can ask for or even think of. This baby that I am asking for is minimal compared to the miracles that he performs every day. I don't want to be the one that gives up on God because he never gives up on me. When God asks a task of me, no matter how long it takes me to do it, no matter how much I mess up, no matter what I do; he's right there. My God has brought people back to life, delivered people out of impossible situations, and he has given barren women the miracle of birthing multiple children. I knew that he could do this small request for me for I am his creation, his friend, and his child.

Some couples dealing with infertility issues may ask, Why Me?  If you are a believer, why not you? You say that you love him and that you are willing to serve him. Sometimes we say we would do anything for him, yet we start giving limitations when times get hard; did you mean it? God does not intend for you to suffer, but when you go through certain situations, it is to build you up. You go through trials so that you can draw closer to God and trust him more. You go through some trials just so that God can get the Glory. My testimony has helped women get through their infertility journey with an easier transition. When I see someone that is going through a similar situation, I share what I have been through. Sharing with others always seems to inspire hope. Women have come back me and said how much my story gave them strength or gave direction for the next step in their process. I know that through this book it will help even more couples.

If I had to go through five years of this infertility journey to help a hundred other couples with their issues and give them encouragement, it was worth the wait. Someone could draw closer to God because of what I went through and how I went through it. That is worth it. If I had to bare this for God's glory, it's worth it. Jesus went through so much more so that I can have an opportunity to have everlasting life. This journey was trivial compared to that. He chose you because you can handle this. Don't give up.

# CHAPTER 8

# For this Child, I Prayed

I connected with a specific story in the bible heavily while I waited for my miracle and that was the story of Hannah. There are a couple of women in the bible who struggled with infertility, but I was fonder of this scripture. For every situation in your life, there is an example in the bible that will parallel to your life's circumstance. The story of Hannah spoke to not only my pain, but it also gave me hope for an expected end. This scripture speaks to women with infertility issues, but it also speaks to the men who support their women with infertility issues.

Hannah's story is found in *I Samuel chapter 1.* I would love you to stop here and read this chapter so that you can fully understand when I reference it. If you are familiar with it, reread it to get a fresh revelation. Yes, Read the whole chapter.

******************

In short, Elkanah had two wives Peninnah and Hannah. Peninnah had children and Hannah did not. Elkanah would make his yearly offering to God. He would offer a piece of his sacrificial meat to Peninnah and the kids, but he gave Hannah a double portion. Year after year Peninnah would taunt Hannah about inability to have kids just to irritate her; it worked. Hannah would cry and she would refuse to eat. Elkanah asked her, "why are you crying and why are you not eating?" He said, "am I not better than ten sons?" She went to the temple of the lord to pray, and the bible said she was in a bitterness of soul. She prayed, asked the Lord to look upon her affliction, and she asked the Lord not to forget her. She described herself in a sorrowful spirit. She prays and pours herself before the Lord. After she prays, Eli the priest tells her to go in peace. She leaves, eats, and is no longer miserable.

This scripture spoke to me not only because Hannah had a problem conceiving, but also because there are various emotions on display in this chapter. This scripture shows that people in the bible had feelings. Hannah is dealing with some of the same emotions I have identified with at some point on a weekly basis. If you are having infertility issues or have had an infertility issue, there has probably been a Peninnah in your life at some point. We also get to see the husband, Elkanah shows his emotions! Everyone's cards are on the table and I get to identify with these people.

Let's deal with Peninnah first. She is thirsty for attention and she is a hater. That sums her up. She has the life, the kids, and the husband; yet she is still missing something. She may have Elkanah's hand in marriage, but she does not have his heart. On some level, she knows she does not possess his heart and this is why she is acting in such poor taste.

She recognizes that Hannah is the apple of his eye, so she is jealous.

Peninnah has a void and instead of dealing with her issues, she takes it out on Hannah. Out of her emptiness, comes taunting Hannah about not having kids, which is cruel and unnecessary. I can only imagine the words she must have uttered to this woman who was already hurting. Peninnah's disparaging words was like picking at a new scab. The taunting hurt Hannah, but Peninnah's taunting did not accomplish what she intended it to do. She thought she could break Hannah, but instead, it pushed Hannah to change her position. The new position was a position of prayer. This pushed Hannah to pray as if she has never prayed before. You may not like Peninnah, but she is necessary. Now and then, we need an extra boost (negative or positive) to change our position in life.

Elkanah loves his wife Hannah considerably; he shows this love to her with his offerings. Elkanah gives to her because he loves her; and since he adores her, she is given the bigger portion. He checks on her when she is not doing well and tries to comfort her. Hannah's inability to conceive children has not changed his love and affection towards her. If Elkanah could hand her the world, he would. Men, there is no manual for how to deal with infertility issues in your relationship. There will be days when your woman feels like a wreck, and there is nothing you can do to change that. On those days, just be there. Elkanah kept his presence present; he was there for her. That is so important; show her you care. Buy that candy bar she likes, get her that dress she likes, surprise her with a date night, leave her a love note in her seat, tell her she is beautiful, wash her car, listen to her, and love on her. Let her know that no matter what happens, you want her and you support her. If she is researching tips to get pregnant, jump on google and help her. Show her that you are in this together. If she gets frustrated, love her anyway. Let her know you are not going anywhere. Women recognize and reward his efforts verbally and physically when he is doing a great job supporting you (so he can keep it going). This is not just your infertility issue or her infertility issue; this issue belongs to both of you. Help each other through it; you are a team.

Then we have Hannah, who is transparent in this scripture. Hannah not only dealt with the void of not having a child, but also endured the taunting from Peninnah. She was already forced to look upon Peninnah with all these kids and endure the slicing of her words constantly. Consequently, people fail to realize that words do not just come out once when are spoken; hurtful words are released and they can replay in the mind repeatedly. Even when Peninnah wasn't around, her words were. Her words cut

Hannah deeply because it was concerning her heart's desire. The Bible shows that Hannah cried. This is a real symptom of longing. I needed to see her go through that. I want to know that when I cry about my desire for a baby, that I was not the only one feeling this way. She stopped eating because she was in a desperate position. She describes herself as bitter, and she describes her condition as an affliction. Some versions of the bible say that she was grieved! To me, this was the perfect word to describe what longing for a child is like, grief.

Moreover, another reason why I love this scripture is because it's not just a sad story. Hannah claims victory in the end. This ending gives hope. The God that I serve today is the same God that Hannah served then. If God did it for her, certainly he loves me enough to do it for me. Hannah took her grief, her tears, her memories of being taunted, and her sorrowful soul to the temple of God and she prayed. She prayed like she never prayed before. Broken and in pieces, she came to God. She was desperate for results. When she left the temple after prayer, she left it all in God's hands.

Feeling better, Hannah left the temple. After she prayed, she stopped crying, and she was able to eat. After she prayed, she was free to worship God! She prayed all the weight off herself. Prayer is essential in this journey through infertility. Prayer gives you strength and lifts weights. Prayer keeps you connected to God and it moves God on your behalf. What else can you do? If you could have fixed the problem, you would have done so by now. Go to God. You may say I have tried prayer before; my response would be to keep trying. Pray until something happens. Pray until something breaks loose. Pray until you see something shifts. Keep praying. You cannot lose with prayer. It is free, and you have everything to gain.

In verse 19, it shows us that they rose up in the morning early, worshipped before the Lord. They returned, and Elkanah knew Hannah his wife (they had sex), and the Lord remembered her. After all those years, the Lord remembers her. In verse 20, she conceives. God sees all that you are going through. He hears the words that people speak to you and what they utter about you. He sees the tears you have cried. He knows how bad you want this baby. I am here to remind you that God has not forgotten you. If God remembered Hannah, he will not forget about you. One of my favorite scriptures is verse 27. "For this child, I prayed, and the Lord hath given me my petition which I asked of him." If you face issues with infertility, God loves you. He still answers prayers. Grab this scripture, type it up, and paste it in places that you will see it throughout the day for encouragement: in your car, on your computer monitor, at your desk, in a notebook, and/or on the fridge. You must stay encouraged.

# Chapter 9

# Dear Family and Friends

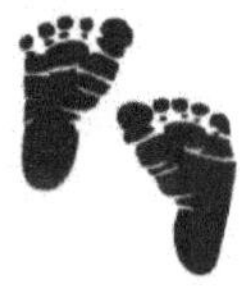

There are people in your life that will truly be there for you when circumstances do not go as planned. Then, there are those that attempt to gain from your pain. There are also those in between people, you know the ones who think they are supportive, but insist on making things harder than have to be. Figure out who is there for you for real, and keep them close. Your support system will lift you up on the days when you are unable to lift yourself up. Be honest, we all have times like this. It is acceptable to lean on people when you need them.

My husband has been there so many days to pick me up even on days when he was hurting himself. He reminded me that God is able to do all things and that he would not lie to us. He reminded me of other blessings God completed in our lives. I also had friends who encouraged me along the way. Sometimes they did not need to say a word, but just listened to me. There were also friends who supported me while managing their own infertility issues simultaneously. They were in the same boat that I was in, and we just continued to lift each other up. The words they said to me often meant so much since I knew that they felt the same feelings that I was feeling. I did not desire for any of my friends or family to be in this situation, but it made me feel better knowing I was not in this battle alone. There is security knowing that others are praying with you and for you. Some people could not relate to what we were going through, but they wanted to see the manifestation of God in our lives because they knew where our hearts were.

During my time battling with infertility, I had a friend who not only encouraged me, but she prayed for me. She also dealt with her issues with the inability to conceive. As she prayed for me, I prayed for her. This gave me an added purpose. She also gave me daily prayers to say specifically for getting pregnant as she said the same prayer for herself. We exchanged stories of disappointment when days were tough, but we also lifted each other right back up in spirit with the word of God.

Not everyone in your life is that refreshing to be around during infertility issues. Often times people don't have ill intention towards you, but they still make you feel inadequate. They ask things like, are you pregnant weekly? Do you have something to tell me? Is there good news yet? Hurry up and have another baby! They may be giddy with excitement for you or just intrusive, but either way, it is not always what you want to face. Due To the longevity of my trial, after a while, the mention of those questions would make my heart sink. Some people even asked me several times a week if I was pregnant.

Between all the people that I encountered in my life, I was consistently faced with this question and answer dance. It becomes a burden. The people asking the questions don't mean for their questions to be a burden, but it is. This message extends to mothers, fathers, grandparents, friends, neighbors, church member, and anyone else who thinks they can just say what they want to you. No matter your relationship with the mother or father to be, sometimes when you make comments relating to conception or lack thereof, it hurts.

## What Not to Say

On behalf of people that struggle with infertility issues, I would like to go over with you what phrases that may come off as inappropriate, may come off mean, or may come off as intrusive when you say them. Please keep in mind that the inflection of your voice matters when saying these phrases as well. These are a culmination of phrases that were said to me or others that I know who also struggled to have children. I know you don't mean any harm, but often times your words hurt. Those that struggle with infertility issues may not say anything to you because they don't want you to be uncomfortable or have your feelings hurt, but saying the following phrases are like small daggers every time they are heard:

1. **You are not pregnant yet?** This makes me feel the pressure of the invisible timetable; as if I missed a deadline somewhere. What you don't know is that I have been trying for months, years, and I missed my own deadline. There is already a level of disappointment that does not need any additional assistance.

2. **What are you waiting for to have a baby (or in my case another baby)?** As if we are just lolly gagging around. The answer to this question is, we are waiting on God. After a few years of getting this, my response was simply "Waiting on God." The conversation is quiet after that.

3. **You can have, borrow, or babysit my kids anytime you want!** Hey, this is no consolation prize for the void I feel. This is not a real solution. This statement won't make anyone feel better.

4. **You other son/daughter needs a sibling!** This may be true, but you telling me this every

time you see me is not speeding this process up.

5. **Is there a Bun in the Oven?** "Yes, right now its unleavened bread" Or "I don't know, do you have a pregnancy test in your purse?" These are things I thought about, but I have never said.

6. **Maybe God has other plans for you?** According to the Holy Bible, this state that I am in is not his perfect plan/will for my life so stop staying that.

7. **Just forget about it, you all are trying too hard**! Can someone who has a disease forget they have a disease? They can't. No matter how much they trust God, they won't forget the fight that they are in, even if they believe they will win. I can't just stop thinking about it. My Bible tells me to procreate, it is commanded by God to procreate, society screams procreate to by a certain age, and there are daily reminders of what I desire all around me. How can I forget? What is trying hard? The thing is that some people don't try at all when they want a baby; it came easy. Once you pass easy street, you make a right onto Try Boulevard, and then a sharp left

onto Try Harder Avenue. If you are trying to get me to relax, this is not helping.

8. **What is taking so long for you to have another one?** Again, this indicates that I missed a deadline. Maybe I missed your deadline. I am sorry that you have been held up by my lazy eggs. Sounds silly right?

9. **Every time you don't feel well, they say, "you must be pregnant".** Or I just have a stomach ache, or I just ate some old seafood, or I am just fatigued. On occasion, people with infertility issues just don't feel well just like other people. Now, due to your comments, you have just given me a compound problem; me thinking about my infertility on top of my temporary illness.

10. **Although this last one is not a phrase, it might as well be. People come up to you and touch your stomach unannounced to feel for the baby that is not growing in your stomach.** This is just rude and wrong. Respect my personal space. If there is no baby there, touching my belly makes me feel worse. I cannot tell you how many times people have done that to me.

A close friend of mine was in a salon getting her nails done and a stranger asked her did she have kids. She responded, "no". The woman then says, "you would never and truly experience womanhood until you have kids". What is that to say? She has no idea why my friend does not have kids. I could not believe someone would say this to anyone, let alone a stranger. Please understand, having children or not having them does not define you! If you do not have children, this does not make you fragment.

Note: It is better to not say anything at all when you don't know what to say. Saying these things above only make it worse. Sometimes it's just better to listen. What is needed at all the times is the prayers of the righteous and/or you can offer an old fashion hug. Moreover, encouragement to keep fighting and believing is always welcomed, and a listening ear is a plus.

# Chapter 10

# The Promise

Getting the call from Dr. Singleton that I finally had conceived was overwhelming. I was so elated. I knew that it would happen one day, but at that moment, I did not know what to do with my emotions. There was someone growing inside of me. I immediately realized that I was carrying a secret around. It was a breathtaking event that left me elated and I couldn't tell anyone about it immediately. After hanging up the phone, I began to thank God.

I remember going to see my baby for the first time after a few weeks through an ultrasound. She was only big enough to see a flicker of a heartbeat; just a quick tiny flutter of light on the machine inside a circle of greatness. I thought to myself, this is what fighting for life looks like. Because of this journey, I can literally tell my daughter I fought for her. I can tell that I never gave up on her, and that I tried relentlessly to bring her here. Most importantly, I can tell her how much I wanted her. The ultrasound picture showed a flicker, but I saw love.

The circumstances of my pregnancy allowed me to hear and see my baby more than the typical pregnancies, since we had to keep an eye on the little flicker. I loved that I had so many chances to see and hear her; it was reassuring. I could watch her all day. Every week that I went back, she was healthy and strong. I carried this baby girl in my stomach like a carton of eggs out of the grocery store. I was probably overly cautious the majority of the time because I did not want to crack this expensive and time-consuming egg. During the first couple of weeks of my pregnancy, I had to continue to take progesterone to keep the lining of uterus strong. I was willing to do whatever I needed to do to maintain a healthy environment for the baby.

I know some women who did not skip a beat during their pregnancy. They were never sick, never had pain, could eat whatever they wanted, and then they could go out and run a marathon. I was not that girl. I would vomit without warning and I was very nauseous with morning sickness a greater portion of my pregnancy, so I was on edge. Due to constant nausea and vomiting, the fatigue was worse than normal because I was not really taking in much food. This made the pregnancy not the jollist pregnancy the whole way through. This baby is what I wanted, so I was willing to take the sickness and anything else. I remained grateful for it all, even while vomiting my guts out. I constantly thanked God for the miracle of life inside of me that he allowed me to carry. Babies are a gift, and God trusted me with one.

On March 26, 2016, at about 2 am, I awoke from a strange feeling, like I peed on myself. This feeling was not accompanied with cramps or contractions. I walked to the bathroom, and more liquid fell down my leg. I was afraid to walk anymore, but I could not keep standing in this spot. I looked over at my husband sound asleep and I decided to keep walking to the bathroom. I sat on the toilet, but nothing came out. I walked back to the bed then more liquid came. By now, I have figured out that this is related to the baby and I was not responsible for peeing myself at age 30. What a relief! However, I don't exactly know what I should do next. In the movies when a woman's water breaks it is not in squirts, it's normally a huge gush of water that drops on the floor. When I had my son, my water was broken in the hospital so I did not have a point of reference that I could tap into. So why is this happening this way? Is this really my water breaking? I tried to wake my husband, but he muttered something ridiculous and went back to sleep. I pondered what to do and waited about fifteen minutes before waking him completely up.

When my husband really woke up, I don't think he took me very seriously. He did see the "pee stains" in the bed, so he knew something happened. We tried to brainstorm the best we could at that hour of the morning; we called the free nurse line at the hospital. They advised us to come to the hospital as soon as possible, but she did not sound concerned. Even after that call, we had no idea what was going on. We knew that we needed to make it to the hospital as directed, so I waddled into the emergency room with a towel between my legs holding it on both sides like a diaper. I did not want to drip all over the place while I was walking in. For some reason, I thought they could plug this liquid up and send me on my merry way. Well, I thought wrong, that did not happen. They wheeled me right upstairs and told me I was having a baby in a few hours. My husband and I were both in shock. This was really happening. She was early. She was not supposed to arrive until sometime in April. They induced my labor slowly over several hours. Once I got to the point of being delirious with pain, she was ready to make her grand entrance.

Did I mention that she was born on the day of her baby shower? While people gathered to play games, eat finger food, and shower me with love, they were surprised to find out that I was a no-show because my daughter was on the way. Not only was she born early; but also during delivery, she did not wait for the doctor. I pushed her right out on the bed just before the doctor sat down to assist me. Here she was, Abigail Daria Shaw born on March 26, 2016, at 4:36 pm at 5lbs 13 ounces and 19 inches. She is proof that it's worth it to wait. She is verification that God keeps his promises. We named her Abigail after my favorite woman in the bible David's wife, Abigail. In the Bible, Abigail was intelligent, resourceful, and her boldness saved many lives including her own. Abigail means Father's Joy in Hebrew and her birth has brought joy in a twofold nature; she has brought joy to God and her father Tyrone. I thank God for trusting me with this test and trusting me with his promise.

My beautiful baby girl Abigail is one and a half years old now. She is very busy, full of personality, strong, extremely smart, and healthy. Her hobbies include watching nursery rhyme shows on Netflix, listening to nursery rhymes music, dancing to nursery rhymes, eating, climbing on top of everything, and she loves licking anything in her sight. She wakes up daily with a smile and is genuinely a happy and fun toddler. The best thing that I love about her personality is that she is very affectionate. She loves hugs and kisses. She even loves to see other people hug or kiss, it makes her giggle. I love her so much, and she was definitely worth everything I had to go through to see her beautiful face.

# Chapter 11

# Prayer

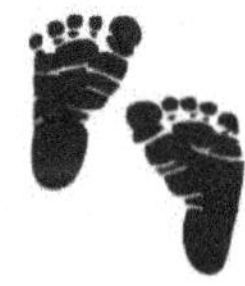

One of the biggest reasons that this infertility journey did not take me out and did not cause me to lose my mind is because of prayer. Yes, prayer. I prayed for myself, my family and I would pray together, my husband prayed for me, my Pastor prayed for me, I linked with others and we prayed together, and others prayed for me. In situations as sensitive and heavy as infertility, prayer has been my safety net. Just like a real safety net, it is there all the time if you set it up and when you need it most, it saves you from harm. Prayer gives me a place to go and be completely naked with God about what I feel and what I need. Prayer time is a time to allow God to guide me through a situation. It is a time for building myself up in faith and building my relationship with God.

It is easy not to pray when life is going great, but that is the time to pray the hardest so that you can stockpile. There will be days when you feel so weak and tired that you can't pray. This is when that back stockpile of prayers will begin to hold you up along with the prayers of others. Surround yourself with people that will pray with you and for you. At my lowest times, I felt prayer lifting me up and getting me through the day. I don't know who it was, or what they said, or how it was keeping me, but the important part was that they took the time to pray for me.

Are you new to prayer? What if you do not know how to pray? You can start today. Prayer is a tool you need. Google about it, read about it, ask someone to teach you. Guess what, prayer does not have to be fancy. God just wants to hear from you. Come as you are to him. What if you are not a believer in this Jesus stuff? You have gone through this so far alone, and nothing has worked, right? Try something new, you have nothing to lose and everything to gain. He can help you get through this. Because prayer is so important, I want to include one here that you can use. Make a copy of this page and put this prayer everywhere. Say it until you have it in your heart and you no longer need a paper.

# *Prayer*

Lord Jesus, I come to you this day to tell you thank you. I thank you for life, health, and strength. I ask that you forgive me of every sin known and unknown. Father, forgive me for anything that I have done knowingly or unknowingly to my body that has caused bareness. Help me to learn to forgive myself for those decisions that were not pleasing to your sight and caused harm to my body. Father, I need you now. I ask that you give me strength. Help me to complete this journey in a way that brings Glory to your name. I pray that you will touch my womb and heal it of any infirmity that causes me not to produce. God, you have called me to be fruitful and multiply, I ask that you line my body up with your word. Father, God, I loose prosperity of healing in my body and throughout my reproductive system. Father, touch my mind right now. Help me to keep my mind stayed on you so that you can keep me in perfect peace while I wait for you to bless me with a child. I declare that depression will not reside in me.  I pray for my spouse, Father that any issue causing my spouse not to produce will be cast down in the name of Jesus. I pray that you will surround my spouse and I with supportive family and friends who will be sensitive to our circumstances and that will pray with us. Father God, I know that by Jesus stripes I am healed. I declare victory over infertility, miscarriages, and bareness. God, I thank you for your grace and your mercy. Father, I praise you in advance for the blessing of this healthy child. I ask you all these things in Jesus name, Amen!

This prayer is something you can say daily. You can add things to it that are specific to your situation. You can take things out that don't pertain to you. This is just a guide. Personalize this prayer. I know by adding this step into your life, it will increase your strength while you wait.

# Passing Seasons

*For the words, I will never say*
*and the things just left unsaid.*
*For the stream of endless thoughts*
*that roundabout my head.*
*For the bottled up frustrations*
*and the things left for not.*
*For the words once unwritten,*
*too discrete to come out.*
*For the secrets that hide within me*
*that strain a quiet shout.*

*When I dig and dig to release,*
*my thoughts then go scurry about.*
*For the imprisoned emotions*
*endowed to the past.*
*For the moments lost in time*
*Now debris or just outcaste.*

*Yellow leaves for changes.*
*Just as seasons tell time.*
*Tears left for water*
*And truth left for lies.*
*Regret so frequently engaged*
*and common are the sighs.*
*Gather a day further*
*those things I dare not say.*
*For the words so far spoken*
*Go back into your cage.*

*And take those feelings with you*
*They have no place to stay.*
*Dungeon those skeletons*
*you hide so deep within.*
*And take that water with you*
*Tears have no place here.*
*Winter soon be nearer so I will hibernate away.*
*For when spring comes*
*I will spring up in a new way!*

**This poem was written from the place of temporary self-imposed isolation. Sometimes you just don't want to burden others down with your temporary emotions. You know that it will pass and you just need a moment; and in those moments, I write. From the encounters from the day situations to the things that people have said, to the things that I saw; they all can overwhelm you. These words were my internal, momentary release. Writing was the only way that I knew how to express myself at a time when the situation seemed bigger than me. After it was written, I pick myself right back up. Defeat can never take up residence inside of me.

# Notes

# Notes

# **Acknowledgements**

Thank you to my loving Husband for loving me without condition. Growing with you and building this family has been my biggest joy. I am grateful to have someone who supports all my dreams and assist me in making my goals reality. This is just the beginning.

To my son Amir, your prayers helped me push through some tough days. Thank you for being such a great big brother. You are sweet, handsome, intelligent, and the best son I could ask for.  I love you.

Aunt Sharon Mckie: For showing me, a taste of what the world has to offer physically and mentally. For sacrificing, for every lesson you embedded in me, for caring for me like your own… Thank you!

Thank you to Pastor Melvin and Evangelist Kathy Wright for praying for me. Thank you for encouraging me and helping me to grow. Thanking you Pastor for pushing and stretching me!

To Apostle Emily Shaw- Drayton, thank you for your Son, for helping me see past myself, for introducing me to Jesus like never known before and for teaching me that Everybody is Somebody.

To Stacey James and Lacey Mack. Thanks for always holding me up and being my voice of reason in every area of my life. You are my sisters, and I love you.

Thank you to Melvina Carpenter for showing me that my dreams don't have to be dreams and for praying with me.

Thank you the late Ms. Reanell Bradley and to my grandparents Dorothy Slater, Sam Miller, Beatrice Praylou, and the late Catherine Hickman for the care you took with me, for the confidence you instilled in me, and for the love you shared with me.

Thank you, Tariekh Henry, for assisting in raising me. When I needed you most, you were there.

To my brother Timothy Battles, I Love you.

To All my former teachers of LCHS thank you. To Mr. Terry Slater and Mrs. Johnson McKnight thank you for exposing me things that don't come in books. What you gave me lives in me daily.

To James Dellinger thank you for not giving up on me, I am so grateful to have a dad like you. Thanks for your continual support in every area of my life. Thank you for being a great Poppa to my children.

Thanks to all my beta readers for all your feedback. Beth Boyce, Rachel Myers, Lacey Mack, Darlene Dellinger, Tyrone Shaw, and to Tara Jordan helping with editing.

# Resources

The Fertility Center of Charleston with Dr. Stephanie Singleton (my doctor) located in Mt. Pleasant South Carolina and there is a location in Savannah Georgia.

There are support groups on Facebook for people who are having infertility issues such as <u>Circle + Bloom Infertility Support Circle</u>. Pleases infertility in your search engine and many groups will pop up, even some for men. Check your local area for any support groups that hold sessions.

Ovia Fertility Tracker is an electronic app you can download on google playstore. *Taking Charge of Your Fertility* by Toni Weschler, MPH taught me about my body. Every woman needs this book.

Here are a few websites below that can help with infertility issues, resources, financial barriers, support group, and more. Some of these sites even give you information on financing fertility treatment through grants and scholarships.

www.Resolve.org                     www. Arcfertility.com

www.ihr.com                         www.fertilitylifelines.com

yourfertilityhub.com

# Bibliography

## Introduction

<u>www.cdc.gov/reproductivehealth/index</u>, p. 8

## Chapter 5

<u>www.Americanpregnancy.org/infertility/male-infertility</u>, p. 42

## Chapter 8

Holy Bible. New King James Version. I Samuel Chapter 1, p. 63-68

# ABOUT THE AUTHOR

Anita Shaw is a Disability Examiner for Vocational Rehabilitation and a Minister in her local ministry. Anita and her husband Tyrone have two beautiful children Abigail and Amir. They currently live in Charleston, South Carolina. In 2007, Anita graduated from Charleston Southern University with her B.S. in Psychology and Sociology. She graduated in 2012 from Capella University with an M.S. in Human Services, with a concentration in Counseling Studies. She has worked in the Human Service field for the State of S.C. for nine years. She loves spending time with her family, writing, traveling, and more importantly, she loves God. This is her first book. Being an published author has been her dream since she was a little girl and she hopes that her words inspire and encourage others.

I invite you to like my Facebook page ASHAWBOOKS.
Drop by and leave your comments about the book or
just share your story.
I would love to hear from you!
Like me on IG: A.SHAWBOOKS


Email me at  a.shawbooks@yahoo.com


Books can be purchased at Amazon.com.
**Please take a few moments to leave your review.**


**Thank you for support!**

Lastly, on the front cover is a very special baby. Her name is **Adelle James**. I chose her picture for the cover because like me, her mother struggled with infertility. She was told by doctors that she wouldn't be able to ever have children. Adelle is further proof that at age 1, God has the final say.